THE 7-DAY ENERGY SURGE

The 7-Day Energy Surge

Boost Your Vitality Naturally

B. VINCENT

QuillQuest Publishers

Contents

Introduction: Unleashing Your Natural Energy

In the present speedy world, where the requests of day to day existence frequently leave us feeling depleted and exhausted, tracking down maintainable ways of supporting our energy levels has never been more significant. The 7-Day Energy Flood: Lift Your Imperativeness Normally isn't simply an aide; it's a groundbreaking excursion intended to revive your life from the back to front. This book intends to furnish you with the devices and information important to open a wellspring of normal energy, upgrading your general prosperity and empowering you to make every second count.

Energy is the pith of life. The crucial power drives our everyday exercises, fills our interests, and supports our fantasies. However, large numbers of us depend on transitory fixes to battle exhaustion, from caffeine-loaded refreshments to caffeinated drinks, uninformed about the regular and manageable options available to us. Truly, the way in to an enduring energy flood lies not in that frame of mind of espresso but rather inside the actual texture of our way of life decisions — from the food sources we eat and the examples of our rest to our active work and mental prosperity.

This book is conceived out of the comprehension that imperativeness ought not be a slippery state, held for the rare sorts of people who appear to have an interminable inventory of energy. All things being equal, it is a feasible reality for everybody, paying little mind to progress in years or foundation. Through a cautiously organized 7-day plan, we will investigate the complex way to deal with supporting your energy normally. Every day will zero in on a particular subject — detoxing, diet, work out, rest, stress the executives, social associations, and manageability — made to expand upon the past, finishing in a far reaching technique for supported essentialness.

Be that as it may, why normal strategies? The response is basic: what we look for isn't simply a flashing spike in energy yet a significant, enduring change by they way we feel and capability. Normal strategies, established in age-old insight and upheld by current science, offer an agreeable way to accomplishing this change, adjusting our bodies and psyches to the rhythms of life that advance wellbeing, bliss, and energy.

As we leave on this excursion together, recollect that the objective isn't flawlessness however progress. The 7-day plan is intended to be a beginning stage, an impetus for long haul change in your way to deal with wellbeing and energy. By making little, sensible changes in your day to day schedules and propensities, you'll start to see critical enhancements in your energy levels, state of mind, and generally speaking wellbeing.

In this way, whether you're hoping to conquer the mid-evening droop, work on your actual perseverance, or just wake up feeling revived and prepared to require on the day, The 7-Day Energy Flood is your manual for a more lively, fiery life. How about we set out on this excursion together, with receptive outlooks and hearts, prepared to open the unlimited energy that nature has coming up for us.

Chapter 1

Chapter 1: Understanding Energy and Vitality

What is Imperativeness?

Imperativeness is something other than the shortfall of weariness; it addresses a complete condition, including actual strength, mental clearness, close to home versatility, and a lively soul. This unique energy pushes us forward, empowering us to connect completely with life's chances and difficulties. Imperativeness enables us to awaken feeling invigorated, tackle our day with energy, and end our night with a feeling of achievement and happiness.

At its center, imperativeness is about balance. It's

the amicable working of our physical and intellectual capacities, making a feeling of wellbeing and aliveness. This condition of balance permits us to perform at our best, no matter what the job that needs to be done, be it proficient obligations, proactive tasks, or taking part in imaginative and social undertakings.

Wellsprings of Energy: The Organic Viewpoint

Energy creation in the human body is a wonder of nature, a complicated cycle that energizes each thought, development, and heartbeat. The foundation of this cycle is the mitochondria, small organelles tracked down in pretty much every cell. These minuscule forces to be reckoned with convert supplements from our food into adenosine triphosphate (ATP), the essential energy transporter in every single living organic entity. The effectiveness of this transformation cycle straightforwardly impacts our energy levels and in general essentialness.

A few key elements influence mitochondrial capability and, likewise, our energy creation:

Supplement admission: The nature of our eating regimen straightforwardly influences mitochondrial productivity. Supplements like magnesium, omega-3 unsaturated fats, and cell reinforcements support mitochondrial wellbeing, while an eating regimen high in handled food varieties and sugars can weaken capability.

Oxygen supply: Customary active work expands the limit of our blood to convey oxygen and improves the respiratory proficiency of our cells, the two of which are significant for ideal mitochondrial execution.

Poison openness: Ecological poisons and stress can harm mitochondria, prompting diminished energy creation. Limiting openness and improving our body's detoxification processes are fundamental for keeping up with essentialness.

Factors Influencing Energy Levels

Understanding the complex idea of energy is significant. A few key elements impact our imperativeness, each connecting with and influencing the others in complex ways:

Rest: Maybe the most essential component of energy and imperativeness, rest is the point at which the body goes through fix and recovery. The quality and amount of rest essentially influence our mental capability, close to home equilibrium, and actual wellbeing. Profound, helpful rest is fundamental for the body to deliver development chemical, fix tissues, and solidify memory.

Sustenance: The maxim "the type of food you eat will affect you general health" turns out as expected with regards to energy and essentialness. A decent eating regimen wealthy in entire food sources gives the supplements important to ideal energy creation and cell wellbeing. Alternately, slims down high in refined sugars, undesirable fats, and counterfeit added substances can prompt vacillations in energy levels and add to long haul medical problems.

Active work: Normal activity improves cardiovascular wellbeing, helps mitochondrial productivity, and increments endorphin levels, adding to an increased feeling of energy and prosperity. Both high-impact and obstruction preparing assume basic parts in keeping up with and further developing our energy levels.

Stress The board: Persistent pressure can exhaust our energy holds, prompting weakness and diminished imperativeness. Figuring out how to oversee pressure through strategies like care, contemplation, and breathing activities can assist with saving our energy and improve our flexibility.

Hydration: Satisfactory hydration is fundamental for all physical processes, including energy creation. Indeed, even gentle lack of hydration can prompt weariness, diminished mental capability, and impeded actual execution.

Social Associations: The nature of our social co-operations and connections can fundamentally affect our energy levels. Positive, steady connections can upgrade our essentialness, while poisonous or depleting connections can drain it.

By tending to every one of these areas, we can adopt an all encompassing strategy to helping our energy levels and upgrading our essentialness. The interconnectedness of these elements implies that upgrades in a single region frequently lead to benefits in others, making a positive pattern of energy improvement.

As we dive further into the 7-Day Energy Flood plan, we will investigate explicit procedures and practices in every one of these areas to assist you with accomplishing a critical lift in your essentialness. From streamlining your eating regimen and work-out everyday practice to working on your rest and overseeing pressure, every day of the arrangement is intended to expand upon the last, finishing in a far reaching way to deal with renewing your energy and upgrading your general prosperity.

Remain tuned as we set out on this excursion to open the key to regular imperativeness and find the energetic energy that exists in you.

Chapter 2

Chapter 2: The 7-Day Energy Surge Plan

Setting out on the excursion to support your imperativeness normally includes an exhaustive arrangement that addresses all parts of prosperity. The 7-Day Energy Flood Plan is intended to launch your excursion toward supported energy levels through designated everyday activities zeroing in on diet, work out, rest, stress the board, and that's just the beginning. This section frames the all-encompassing construction of the arrangement, setting you up for the extraordinary week ahead.

Outline of the 7-Day Plan

The arrangement is organized around everyday subjects, each structure on the last, to slowly present propensities and practices that add to a flood in energy and generally speaking essentialness. The objective isn't simply to feel an impermanent lift in energy however to establish the groundwork for maintainable way of life changes that keep on delivering profits in essentialness and wellbeing long after the underlying week has passed.

Day 1: Detox and Purify centers around taking out poisons and diminishing aggravation through diet and hydration, making way for upgraded energy creation.

Day 2: Invigorating Through Diet presents supplement thick food varieties that are known to support energy levels, zeroing in on adjusting macronutrients to productively fuel your body.

Day 3: Fueling Up with Exercise coordinates actual work that invigorates energy creation, utilizing a blend of cardiovascular, strength, and adaptability works out.

Day 4: Reestablishing with Rest focuses on further developing rest quality, underlining schedules and conditions that advance peaceful rest.

Day 5: Overseeing Pressure tends to the energy channel brought about by pressure, presenting procedures for stress the board and profound prosperity.

Day 6: Association and Social Imperativeness investigates the empowering force of social associations and local area, offsetting social exercises with time for isolation and reflection.

Day 7: Supporting Your Energy Flood centers around techniques for keeping up with and expanding upon the week's force, defining objectives, and anticipating long haul essentialness.

Every day, you will be directed through unambiguous exercises, dietary suggestions, activities, and unwinding procedures customized to the subject, intended to be sensible yet effective.

Planning for the Energy Flood

Before you plunge into Day 1, a little planning can guarantee your prosperity over time and then some. This arrangement includes mental, physical, and calculated viewpoints to embrace the arrangement completely.

Mental Arrangement:

Set Clear Goals: Consider the reason why you're attempted this excursion. Whether it's to battle weariness, further develop wellbeing, or basically to feel more invigorated, remembering your objectives will inspire you through testing minutes.

Embrace Transparency: Be ready to attempt new food varieties, exercises, and schedules. Receptiveness to change is critical for development and improvement.

Actual Climate Arrangement:

Put together Your Space: Guarantee your living climate upholds your objectives. This could mean cleaning up your kitchen to account for solid concocting or setting a happy with, welcoming space for exercise and contemplation.

Prep Your Storage room: Stock up on the food varieties and drinks you'll require, zeroing in on new, entire fixings and taking out allurements that could wreck your advancement.

Vital Supplies:

Food and Sustenance: Buy or plan to buy new vegetables, natural products, lean proteins, and entire grains. Hydration will be vital, so more than adequate water and natural teas are likewise fundamental.

Gym equipment: While many activities recommended should be possible with body weight alone, having a yoga mat, opposition groups, or light loads can improve your experience.

Unwinding Helps: Things like natural balms, a diary for reflection, and any contemplation helps can uphold your pressure the board and rest improvement endeavors.

Making way for your 7-Day Energy Flood is about something beyond sticking to the script; it's tied in with starting a change in your way of life and prosperity. With your expectations clear and your current circumstance prepared, you're prepared to set out on this excursion to normally help your imperativeness. We should push ahead with reason, excitement, and an open heart to the vast potential outcomes that a flood in energy can bring to our lives.

Chapter 3:
Day-by-Day
Guide

Day 1: Detox and Purify model

Wake-up routine

Warm Lemon Water

Start your energy flood venture with a straightforward yet significant custom: a glass of warm lemon water after waking. This drink goes about as a delicate reminder for your stomach related framework, assisting with flushing out poisons, launch your digestion, and alkalize your body. The L-ascorbic acid from the lemon helps your invulnerable framework, setting up your body and psyche for the day ahead.

Delicate Yoga Arrangement

Take part in a 15-minute delicate yoga grouping

intended to animate your stomach related framework and improve blood course. Focus on represents that turn and pack the mid-region, as situated wind and feline cow extends, to help the body's normal detoxification process. This careful activity establishes a quiet vibe for the afternoon, zeroing in on inside purging and mental clearness.

Breakfast: Green Detox Smoothie

Set up a supplement rich green smoothie for breakfast. Consolidate spinach for its elevated degrees of iron and magnesium, cucumber for hydration, green apple for a sprinkle of normal pleasantness and fiber, ginger for its stomach related advantages, and avocado for sound fats to keep you feeling full and fulfilled. This creation isn't simply feeding yet in addition upholds hydration and fills you with energy, without burdening your stomach related framework.

Early in the day Action: Light Activity

Early in the day, participate in light activity. Decide on a 30-minute stroll in nature or a bouncing back meeting on a smaller than expected trampoline. These exercises are especially viable for invigorating the lymphatic framework, upgrading detoxification, and supporting blood flow, all of which add to expanded energy levels and a positive state of mind.

Lunch: Purging Plate of mixed greens

For lunch, set up a purging plate of mixed greens stacked with blended greens, crude vegetables like carrots and beets, and a basic lemon-olive oil dressing. This feast is loaded with cell reinforcements, fiber, and fundamental supplements, supporting the detoxification interaction while giving a light yet invigorating late morning dinner.

Evening: Natural Coffee Break

In the early evening, pause for a minute for a natural coffee break. Pick teas with detoxifying properties, for example, dandelion or green tea, which support liver wellbeing and give a delicate jolt of energy without a bad case of nerves related with caffeine.

Supper: Steamed Vegetables and Quinoa

Supper on Day 1 ought to comprise of steamed vegetables and quinoa. This mix offers an equilibrium of complicated sugars, protein, and fiber, guaranteeing satiety without substantialness. It's an optimal method for finishing the day's feasts on a light note, supporting for the time being detoxification and rest.

Evening Unwinding: Contemplation

Close your day with a reflection meeting zeroing in on profound breathing to upgrade the body's regular detoxification processes. This training assists with quieting the brain, diminish pressure, and further develop rest quality, which are all significant for revival and energy.

Chapter 4

Chapter 4: Complementary Practices for Sustained Vitality

In the wake of committing seven days to supporting your energy normally, significant to investigate and coordinate corresponding practices guarantee supported essentialness past the underlying flood. These practices are intended to brace the increases made, assisting you with keeping a dynamic, vivacious state in your day to day routine. This part dives into care and reflection, the job of enhancements and spices, and the significance of hydration, giving a comprehensive way to deal with long haul energy the board.

Care and Contemplation

Prologue to Care: Care is the act of being available and completely drew in with anything we're doing right now, liberated from interruption or judgment. This segment presents the idea of care, making sense of its underlying foundations in Buddhist practice and its pertinence in the present high speed world. By developing care, people can diminish pressure and nervousness, further develop concentration and discernment, and upgrade generally speaking prosperity, which straightforwardly influences energy levels.

Contemplation Methods for Energy: Reflection, a critical part of care practice, includes different procedures that can assist with overseeing pressure, further develop rest, and lift energy. This piece of the section guides perusers through basic reflection practices like centered consideration contemplation, where one focuses on a solitary perspective (like breathing), and careful mindfulness rehearses, which include focusing on contemplations and sensations without judgment. The part makes sense of how these procedures can assist with reseting the brain, prompting worked on mental energy and imperativeness.

Enhancements and Spices

Normal Enhancements for Energy: While a fair eating routine is the foundation of supported energy, certain regular enhancements can offer extra help. This fragment covers nutrients and minerals basic for energy digestion, like B-nutrients, iron, magnesium, and Coenzyme Q10 (CoQ10), making sense of their jobs and the advantages of supplementation, especially for people with dietary limitations or explicit ailments.

Invigorating Spices: Spices have been utilized for a really long time to help wellbeing and imperativeness. This segment acquaints perusers with spices known for their energy-helping properties, like ginseng, rhodiola rosea, and ashwagandha. It talks about how these spices can assist with upgrading actual execution, lessen weakness, and further develop pressure flexibility, offering rules for protected and compelling use.

Hydration: The Overlooked Yet truly great individual

Effect of Water on Energy Levels: Water is fundamental forever, yet its significance in keeping up with energy and imperativeness is frequently ignored. This part underscores the job of hydration in energy creation, featuring how even gentle drying out can debilitate actual execution, mental capability, and temperament. It makes sense of the physiological cycles behind these impacts and offers reasonable ways to remain enough hydrated over the course of the day.

Techniques for Improving Hydration: Perceiving the difficulties certain individuals face in polishing off sufficient water, this part gives imaginative and powerful systems to expanding liquid admission. Ideas incorporate implanting water with leafy foods for flavor, setting normal drinking updates, and utilizing applications or water bottles that track admission. It likewise addresses the significance of changing hydration levels in light of action, environment, and individual wellbeing needs.

By integrating these reciprocal practices into their day to day schedules, perusers can not just keep up with the energy flood accomplished during the underlying 7-day plan yet additionally expand upon it, guaranteeing long haul imperativeness and a dynamic, satisfying life.

Chapter 5: Troubleshooting and Overcoming Setbacks

In the wake of leaving on the excursion to support your essentialness normally, you might experience difficulties en route. This part is committed to recognizing normal obstacles and giving pragmatic arrangements, guaranteeing that you can keep up with your freshly discovered energy levels and keep advancing towards ideal wellbeing and imperativeness.

Normal Difficulties and Arrangements

Weariness Regardless of Endeavors: Now and then, even with a decent eating regimen, satisfactory rest, and normal activity, you could in any case feel tired.

This could be because of basic issues like lacks of nutrient, drying out, or stress. Survey your propensities, guarantee you're hydrating adequately, overseeing pressure, and consider a look at up to lead lacks or medical issue.

Battling with Consistency: Keeping up with new propensities can challenge. Assuming that you end up battling to adhere to the 7-day plan or the reciprocal practices, have a go at separating them into more modest, more reasonable advances. Put forth practical objectives, celebrate little triumphs, and recall that advancement, not flawlessness, is vital.

Absence of Inspiration: Inspiration melts away when objectives appear to be far off or challenging to accomplish. Revive your excitement by returning to your explanations behind beginning this excursion. Interface with a local area or track down a pal with comparable objectives to share encounters and consolation. Envisioning the advantages of further developed essentialness can likewise reignite your drive.

Using time effectively: Carving out opportunity for solid propensities is a typical impediment. Review your everyday daily schedule to distinguish time sinks and focus on exercises that add to your energy levels. Arranging feasts, exercises, and unwinding time ahead of time can likewise assist with smoothing out your timetable, making it more straightforward to keep up with your new way of life.

Managing Pressure: Stress is a critical energy drainer. Execute pressure decrease methods like profound breathing activities, care reflection, or yoga into your everyday daily schedule. Perceiving and overseeing stressors proactively can keep them from subverting your energy levels and in general prosperity.

When to Look for Proficient Assistance

Perceiving the Signs: Tireless weariness or an absence of imperativeness, notwithstanding following a sound way of life, may demonstrate hidden medical problems. Side effects to look for incorporate steady weariness, tremendous changes in rest designs, unexplained weight changes, or sensations of melancholy or uneasiness. On the off chance that you experience these side effects, it's fundamental to talk with a medical care proficient to recognize any hidden circumstances.

Looking for Master Guidance: Medical services experts can offer customized exhortation and therapies custom-made to your particular requirements. This might incorporate far reaching wellbeing assessments, healthful guiding, or stress the board techniques. Furthermore, for those with ongoing ailments, proficient direction guarantees that any way of life changes supplement existing treatment plans and backing in general wellbeing. Keep in mind, looking for help is an indication of solidarity and a significant stage in focusing on your wellbeing and imperativeness.

Beating mishaps on your way to expanded energy and essentialness is a necessary piece of the excursion. By recognizing normal difficulties and executing the procedures framed in this section, you can explore these hindrances effectively. Keep in mind, each step in the right direction, regardless of how little, is progress toward a more dynamic, lively life.

Conclusion: Your Path to Lasting Vitality

As we close the pages of "The 7-Day Energy Flood: Lift Your Imperativeness Normally," it's critical to consider the excursion we've left upon together. This guide was planned not similarly as an impermanent lift to your energy levels, yet as a central shift towards a more lively, enthusiastic life. The way to enduring essentialness is both an excursion and an objective, one that requires responsibility, care, and a readiness to embrace change.

All through this book, we've investigated different normal techniques to improve your imperativeness, from detoxifying your body and invigorating through diet, to fueling up with practice and reestablishing your energy through quality rest. We've additionally dove into the significance of overseeing pressure, interfacing with others, and supporting your energy flood with corresponding practices and investigating tips. Every section has offered experiences and note-worthy stages to help you accomplish and keep a condition of high energy and prosperity.

As you push ahead, recollect that essentialness is definitely not a consistent state yet a fluctuating one, impacted by many variables, including your actual wellbeing, close to home equilibrium, and ecological circumstances. There will be days when you feel relentless and others when your energy fades. This is normal and not out of the ordinary. The key isn't to take a stab at flawlessness yet for progress, to gain from difficulties, and to ceaselessly adjust your systems to meet the changing requirements of your body and psyche.

Embrace Change and Observe Progress

Change, while testing, is additionally a chance for development. Embrace the way of life changes you've made during this 7-day venture as steps towards a better, more lively you. Praise your advancement, regardless of how little it might appear. Every positive change is a triumph by its own doing, adding to your general essentialness.

Keep a Comprehensive Methodology

Imperativeness isn't exclusively the result of actual wellbeing; it includes your psychological, profound, and otherworldly prosperity. Keep on supporting all parts of your being, understanding that equilibrium is vital to supporting energy. Integrate care rehearses, support your body with entire food varieties, remain dynamic, interface with friends and family, and set aside a few minutes for rest and unwinding.

Adjust and Change

Your way to imperativeness is remarkably yours,

and what works for you might change over the long haul. Pay attention to your body, and adjust your methodology as the need might arise. Consistently evaluate your energy levels, wellbeing status, and in general prosperity, changing your methodologies to line up with your ongoing necessities and objectives.

Look for Help

Keep in mind, you don't need to walk this way alone. Look for help from companions, family, wellbeing experts, or similar networks. Sharing your encounters, difficulties, and triumphs can give inspiration, motivation, and important experiences.

The Excursion Proceeds

This book denotes the start of your excursion to enduring essentialness, not the end. Every day presents another potential chance to live more vigorously, to embrace life completely, and to splendidly focus your light. Convey forward the illustrations took in, the practices embraced, and the mentality shifts accomplished. Keep on investigating, try, and draw in with life in manners that advance your being and hoist your energy.

Much obliged to you for taking this excursion with me. May the way forward be brilliant, and your energy unlimited. Here's to your wellbeing, bliss, and steadily flooding essentialness.

Appendices

The supplements segment is intended to give you extra assets to help and upgrade your excursion towards supported essentialness. These pragmatic devices incorporate recipes for energy-helping feasts and bites, test work-out schedules, and contemplation and care works out. Every asset is planned to make it more straightforward for you to coordinate the standards and practices examined all through this book into your day to day existence.

Appendix A: Recipes for Energy-Boosting Meals and Snacks

Green Power Smoothie

Spinach (1 cup)

Avocado (1/2, peeled and pitted)

Green apple (1, cored and sliced)

Fresh ginger (1-inch piece)

Lemon juice (from 1/2 lemon)

Water or almond milk (1 cup)

Blend all ingredients until smooth. Enjoy this detoxifying smoothie first thing in the morning to kick-start your day.

Quinoa and Black Bean Salad

Cooked quinoa (1 cup)

Black beans (1/2 cup, rinsed and drained)

Cherry tomatoes (1/2 cup, halved)

Cucumber (1/2 cup, diced)

Red onion (1/4 cup, finely chopped)

Cilantro (1/4 cup, chopped)

Lime juice (from 1 lime)

Olive oil (1 tablespoon)

Salt and pepper to taste

Mix all ingredients in a bowl. This salad is packed with protein and fiber, making it a perfect lunch option.

Almond and Date Energy Balls

Almonds (1 cup)

Dates (1 cup, pitted)

Chia seeds (2 tablespoons)

Coconut flakes (1/2 cup)

Cocoa powder (1 tablespoon, optional)

Process almonds and dates in a food processor until they form a sticky mixture. Add chia seeds and cocoa powder (if using) and pulse to combine. Roll the mixture into balls and coat with coconut flakes. Store in the refrigerator for a quick energy snack.

Appendix B: Sample Exercise Routines

Morning Energizer Routine

Jumping jacks (1 minute)

Dynamic stretches (5 minutes)

Bodyweight squats (15 reps)

Push-ups (10 reps)

Plank (1 minute)

This short routine is designed to wake up your body and boost your energy in the morning.

Stress-Relief Yoga Sequence

Cat-Cow Stretch (1 minute)
Downward-Facing Dog (1 minute)
Child's Pose (1 minute)
Forward Fold (1 minute)
Seated Twist (1 minute each side)

Performing this sequence in the evening can help you unwind and de-stress after a busy day.

Appendix C: Meditation and Mindfulness Exercises

Five Senses Exercise

This care practice includes focusing on your five faculties to ground yourself right now. Burn through one moment on each sense, zeroing in on what you can see, hear, smell, taste, and contact. This training can be particularly useful in snapshots of stress or nervousness.

Guided Visualization for Relaxation

Track down an agreeable situated position and shut your eyes. Envision yourself in a serene setting, like an ocean side or a backwoods. Imagine the subtleties of the climate, zeroing in on the tones, sounds, and aromas. Burn through 5-10 minutes here, permitting yourself to profoundly unwind.

These reference sections offer apparatuses and practices to assist you with supporting the energy flood accomplished through the 7-day plan. By integrating these recipes, activities, and care methods into your daily schedule, you can keep on supporting your essentialness and prosperity long subsequent to finishing the program.